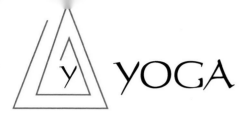

YOGA

Yoga ABC's

Written/Illustrated by Elizabeth C. Kawecki, President/Director of Y Yoga Inc.

JayMar Printing • Richardson, Texas

Cover/Illustrations by Elizabeth C. Kawecki
Copyright 2009
The cataloging-in-publication data on file with the Library of Congress

ISBN 978-0-578-04017-2

Published by Y Yoga Inc.

To order: Y Yoga Inc., 961687 Gateway Blvd., Suite 201E, Amelia Island, FL 32034
www.yyoga.com.
Info@yyoga.com

Disclaimer:
It is recommended that you consult with a licensed medical doctor or physician before commencing any exercise program, especially if you have a medical condition or are pregnant. Neither the author nor the publisher can accept responsibility for, or shall be liable for, any accident, injury, loss or damage (including any consequential loss) that results from using the ideas, information, procedures or advice offered in this book.

This book is dedicated to my nephews
Joey and Jack, my nieces Hannah, Bailey and Gracie.
Their playfulness, vivid imagination and creativity
inspired me to pursue this dream.

This book is my way of sharing my love of yoga with children.
Their vivid imagination, free thinking, playfulness and simplicity
in just being, has been a constant source of joy in my life.
Hopefully, this book will allow children to develop their own
poses or postures (asanas) by playing and moving their
bodies while freeing their minds and igniting their individual spirits.

WHY YOGA / BENEFITS OF YOGA

Why should children do yoga? Yoga is important to children because their lives are sometimes very hectic or stressful. Yoga teaches children to relax, and also provides a great overall workout resulting in the better utilization of the body, the mind, and the breath. There are many other benefits to doing yoga by children.

- Gives a child time to slow down, unwind and work at their own pace in a non-competitive environment.
- Improves a child's flexibility, strength, and balance at the same time enhancing their athletic abilities while preventing injury.
- Develops their ability to learn by not only using both sides of the brain, but all of their senses.
- Helps reinforce a positive body image (correct posture) which builds self confidence and self-esteem.
- Balances emotions through movement and breathing.
- Yoga is FUN; fueling their individual spirit, imagination and creativity, whether it be done alone, with a friend or a group.

BREATHING (PRANAYAMA)

How we breathe is very important. We must learn to breathe properly in order to calm and quiet the restlessness of the mind (main purpose of yoga), while connecting with our body. Breathing correctly relaxes and invigorates the body at the same time.

Begin in INDIAN POSE/PRETZEL POSE/EASY SITTING POSE (SUKANASANA)
Sit on the ground with your spine tall.
Bend your knees and cross your legs.

Try one of the following breaths:

(1) POW WOW BREATH/YOGI BREATH (DEERGHA SWASAM)
HELPS TO FOCUS THE MIND AND STILL THE BODY BEFORE AND AFTER A STRESSFUL ACTIVITY OR SPORTING EVENT, ESPECIALLY WHEN FEELING TENSE.
Place your right hand on your mouth.
Breathe in through your nose. Keep your mouth closed.
Breathe out through your nose.
Place the other hand on your abdomen, center of chest, or below your throat. Feel your breath move.

(2) BUNNY BREATH
PROVIDES A QUICK BURST OF ENERGY TO AWAKEN THE MIND AND BODY DURING THE DAY WHEN FEELING TIRED.
Wrinkling up your nose, sniff three times breathing in through your nose.
Open your mouth and breathe out one breath.

(3) DRAGON BREATH

BALANCES EMOTIONS (LIKE FEELINGS OF ANGER OR FRUSTRATION) WHILE RESTORING ENERGY.

Breathe in through your nose.

Open your mouth wide and breathe out through your mouth exhaling forcefully.

(4) BEE BREATH

HELPS TO CALM AND FOCUS THE MIND WHILE ENERGIZING THE BODY.

Breathe in through your nose.

Open your mouth a tiny bit and breathe slowly out through your mouth.

Feel your lips buzzing like a bee.

(5) BREATH OF FIRE

CLEARS YOUR MIND AND INCREASES AWARENESS.

Breathe in through your mouth.

Exhale forcefully out of your mouth continuously for as long as you like.

Do not worry about the breathing in, it will happen naturally.

See your stomach pulse in and out as you feel the heat of your breath

Aa

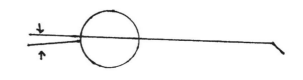

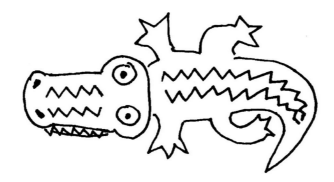

Alligator

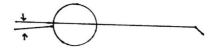

Alligator

**Benefits: slows your heart, eases your breath,
calms your body, stretches your arms**

Lie on your belly on the ground with your legs in a straight line behind you.
Stretch your arms out in front of your ears.
Clap your hands, "chomping" them together.

Bb

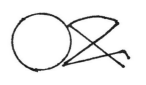

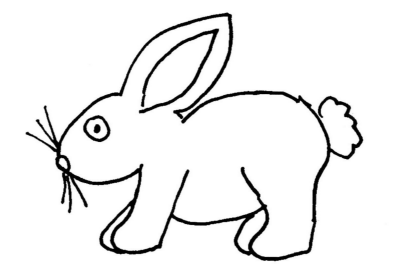

Bunny

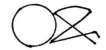

Bunny

Benefits: releases your shoulders and lower back, links your breath and body

Kneel on the ground with your knees and feet together.

Sit on your feet.

Lay your chest and belly on top of your legs.

Put your forehead to the floor.

Tuck your elbows next to your knees.

"Sniff" and wrinkle up your nose.

Hip Hop around like a bunny.

Cc

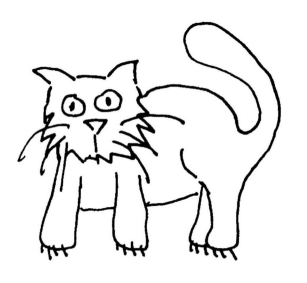

Cat

Cat (Bidalasana)

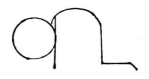

Benefits: works your spine, lets go of tightness in the back, increases blood flow in body

Kneel on the ground with knees under your hips and hands under your shoulders like a table.
Breathe in then drop your chin to your chest.
Round your shoulders to the sky, arching your back like an angry cat.
Pull your belly button in while breathing out.
"Meow" like a cat.
Breathe in and come back to the table position.

Dd

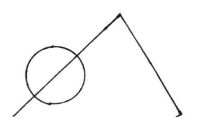

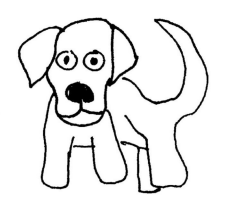

Dog

Dog (Adho Mukha Svanasana)

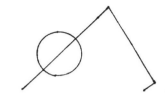

**Benefits: lengthens and strengthens your
arms and legs, quiets your mind**

Kneel on the ground with knees under your hips and hands
under your shoulders like a table.
Curl your toes under.
Lift your bum (tailbone) to the sky as you straighten your legs.
Let your head drop between your arms.
Press your feet downward to the ground, trying to make
your feet flat on the ground.
Wag your tail (bum). "Bark" like a dog.

Ee

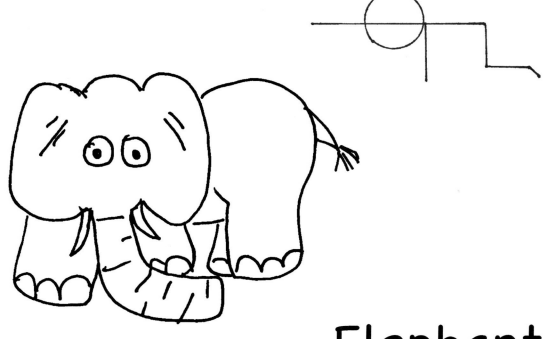

Elephant

Elephant

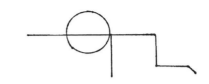

Benefits: stretches your arms and shoulders

Kneel on the ground with your knees under your hips and hands under your shoulders like a table.
Lift your right arm off the ground straight out in front of you.
Swing your arm side to side, swinging your trunk.
Repeat with your left arm.
Make an elephant sound.

Ff

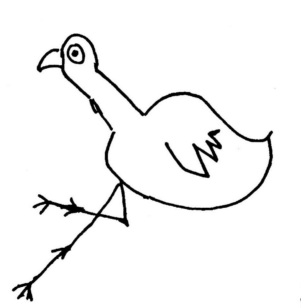

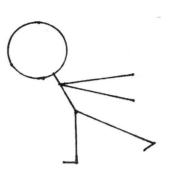

Flamingo

Flamingo

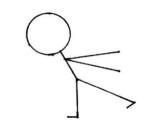

**Benefits: improves your focus, concentration
and balance, strengthens the legs**

Stand tall with your feet lined up under your knees.
Stretch your arms out away from the sides of your body, spreading your wings.
Bend forward from your hips, standing only on your right leg with your foot flat on the ground.
Lift your left leg up behind you toward the sky.
See how long you can stand on one leg.
Repeat with the left foot on the ground and the right leg to the sky.

Gg

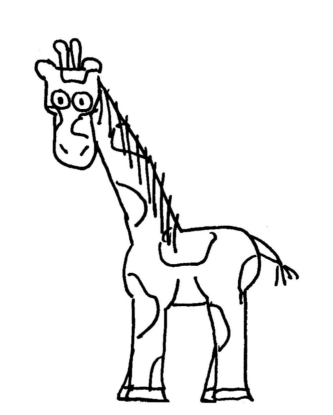

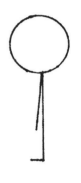

Giraffe

Giraffe

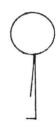

**Benefits: stretches your neck,
lengthens your spine**

Stand tall with your feet together and your arms by your side.
Look up at the sky, lifting your chin away from your chest.

Hh

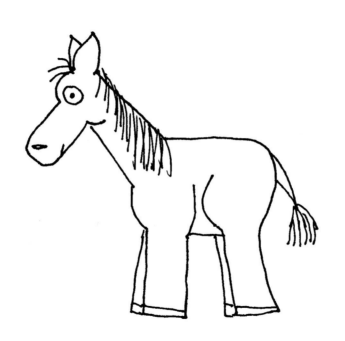

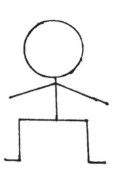

Horse

Horse

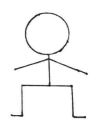

Benefits: opens your hips, stretches and strengthens the front of your legs (quadriceps)

Stand with your feet directly under your shoulders.
Turn your feet out away from your body.
Sit deep dropping your bum toward the ground.
Rock from side to side, galloping.
"Neigh" like a horse.

Ii

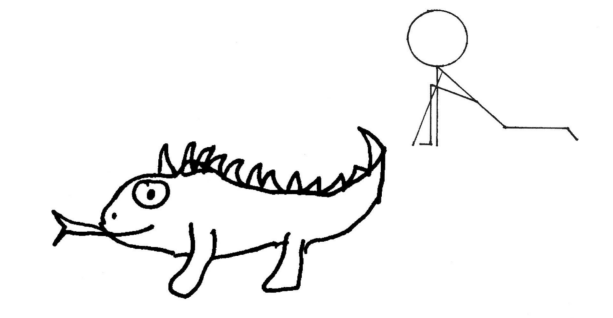

Iguana

Iguana

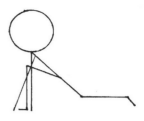

Benefits: opens and stretches the hips

Stand tall with your feet under your knees.
Reach your arms to the sky.
Bend forward from your hips, pushing your bum out.
Bring your hands to the ground.
Step back with your right foot behind. Keep your left foot under your knee.
Drop your right knee to the ground.
Place your left hand to the inside of your left foot.
Slowly bend your elbows lowering your body toward the ground.
Stick your tongue in and out. Blink your eyes.
Repeat stepping your left foot behind. Keep your right foot under knee.

Jj

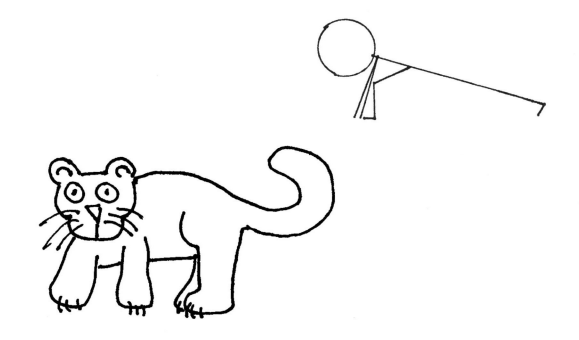

Jaguar

Jaguar

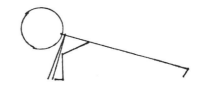

Benefits: stretches your legs and hips

Stand tall with feet under your knees.
Reach your arms to the sky.
Bend forward from your hips, pushing your bum out.
Bring your hands to the ground.
Step back with your right foot. Keep your left foot under your knee.
Step your right foot forward. Bring your right foot back.
Run fast in place by switching your feet back and forth.
"Growl" like a jaguar.

Kk

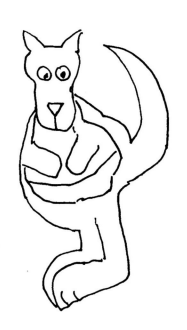

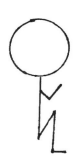

Kangaroo

Kangaroo

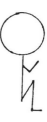

Benefits: strengthens your legs, knees and ankles

Stand tall with your feet and knees together.
Bring your hands together in front of your heart in prayer.
Sit deep, dropping your bum toward the ground and bend your knees.
Hop up and down.

Ll

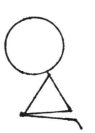

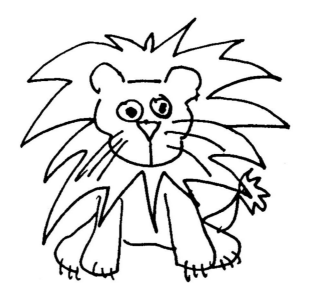

Lion

Lion

Benefits: stretches your ankles, calves and legs

Kneel on the ground with your knees together.
Sit up tall with your bum on your feet.
Put your hands on your knees.
Spread your fingers wide showing your nails.
"Roar"like a lion.
Jump forward and back; lunging to attack.

Silly Lion->stick out your tongue and look up to the sky.

Mm

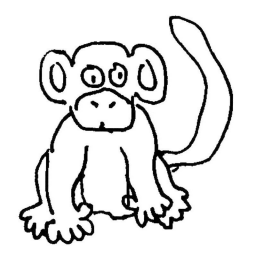

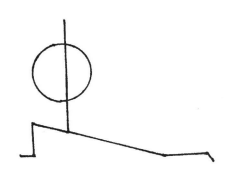

Monkey

Monkey (Hanumanasana)

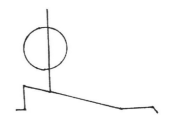

Benefits: stretches your hips, strengthens your knees and ankles, releases your shoulders, works your stomach muscles/belly

Stand tall with your feet under your knees.

Reach your arms to the sky.

Bend forward from your hips, pushing your bum out behind you.

Bring your hands to the ground.

Step back with your right foot back behind you and lower your right knee to the ground. Keep your left foot under your knee.

Straighten your arms to the sky, bringing your palms together.

Make a monkey sound.

Repeat by stepping your left foot back behind you while lowering your left knee to the ground.

Nn

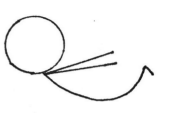

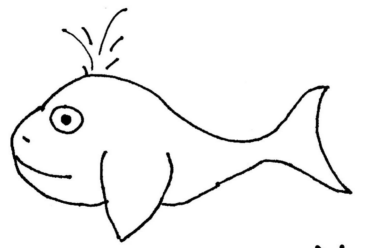

Narwhale

Narwhale

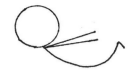

Benefits: releases tightness in your shoulders and upper back, strengthens your entire back

Lie on your belly on the ground with your chin on the floor.
Straighten your arms out by your side away from your body, reaching for your toes.
Bend your knees, lifting your feet off the ground toward your bum.
Press your belly into the ground.
Look up and bring your chin away from your chest.
Lift your chest and arms off the floor, "spouting" water.

Oo

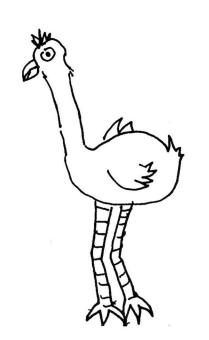

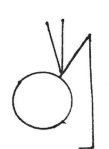

Ostrich

Ostrich

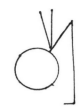

Benefits: stretches your legs, releases tightness in your shoulders, opens your chest, and calms your mind

Stand tall with your feet together and knees in one straight line; keeping your legs straight.
Straighten your arms straight out in front of you.
Bend forward from your hips; pushing your bum out. Bring your hands to touch your toes.
Lift your arms behind you toward the sky, keeping your arms straight.
Hide your head in the sand.

Pp

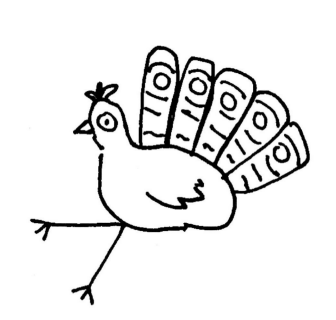

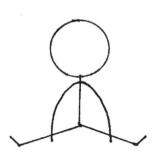

Peacock

Peacock

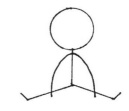

Benefits: stretches your legs, releases tightness in your middle back

Sit up tall on the ground with legs straight out in front of you.
Spread your legs wide.
Straighten your arms and lift them out from your sides away from your body, showing your feathers.
Bend forward from your hips and reach to try to touch the ground between your legs to hide your head in your feathers.

Qq

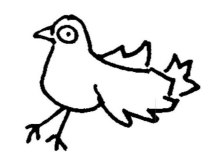

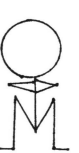

Quail

Quail

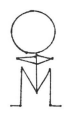

**Benefits: strengthens your hips, knees, ankles
and toes, improves your balance**

Kneel on the ground with your knees apart.
Sit your bum on your feet.
Curl your toes under.
Place your hands on the ground and push back until you are on your toes.
Lift one hand at a time off the ground in front of your heart.
Bring your hands together in prayer.
Bend forward from your hips, putting your elbows to the inside of your knees.
Push your knees away from your body with your elbows, resting your entire body on your toes.

Rr

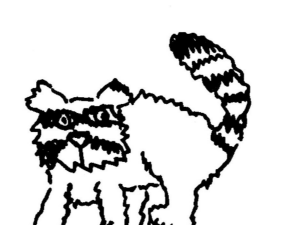

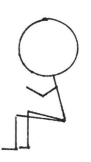

Raccoon

Raccoon

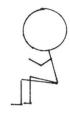

Benefits: strengthens your calves and leg muscles, stretches your arms

Kneel on the ground with your knees apart.
Sit your bum on your feet.
Curl your toes under.
Straighten your arms out in front of you and reach.

Ss

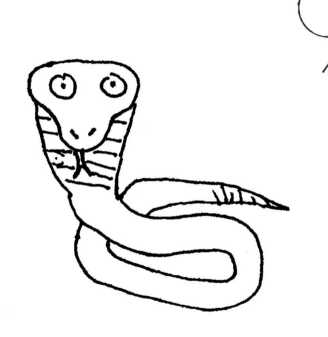

Snake

Snake (Bhujangasana)

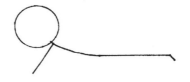

Benefits: opens your chest, strengthens your back, lengthens your spine, increases your blood flow in your body

Lie on your belly on the ground with your feet and legs together.
Put your hands under your shoulders and tuck your elbows next to your ribs or the side of your body.
Look up, lifting your chin away from your chest.
Press your belly and hands into the ground.
Straighten your arms, lifting your chest off the ground.
Stick your tongue out and "hiss" like a snake, moving your hips side to side.

Tt

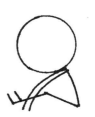

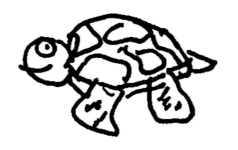

Turtle

Turtle

**Benefits: stretches your legs and lower back,
releases tightness in your shoulders**

Sit up tall on the ground with your legs straight out in front of your body.
Bring the bottom of your feet together with knees out to the side away
from your body.
Slide your hands with the inside of your hands (palms) faced up under your legs.
Drop your head to your toes to hide your head in your shell.

*Suntanning Turtle-> straighten your legs out in front of your body and open your legs wide. Slide your hands
under your legs at or around your knees resting the inside of your hands (palms) on the ground.

Uu

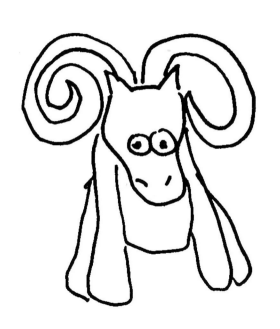

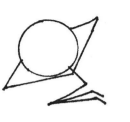

Uriel

Uriel

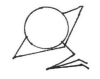

Benefits: stretches your legs, opens your chest,
releases tightness in your shoulders,
strengthens your ankles and knees

Kneel on the ground with your knees touching.
Sit your bum back on your feet.
Place your hands on your head just behind your ears with elbows out away from your body.
Pull your elbows back behind you.
Make a goat sound.

Vv

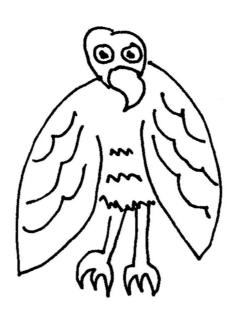

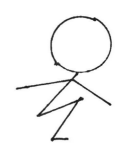

Vulture

Vulture

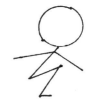

Benefits: strengthens your knees, ankles and toes

Kneel on the ground with your knees apart.
Sit your bum on your feet.
Curl your toes under.
Place your hands on the ground.
Push your body back up straight with your arms, coming onto your toes.
Lift and lower your arms out to your side away from and to your body, flapping your wings.

Ww

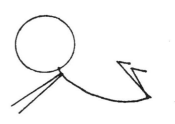

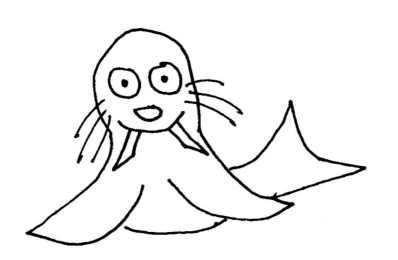

Walrus

Walrus

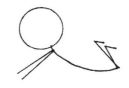

Benefits: strengthens your spine, stretches your arms, shoulders and legs

Lie on your belly on the ground with your chin resting on the ground.
Straighten your legs behind you with legs wide apart.
Straighten your arms out in front ot you.
Push your hands into the ground, lifting your chin, chest and elbows off the ground.
Smile wide showing your teeth (tusks).
Make a walrus sound.

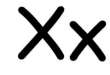

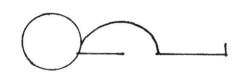

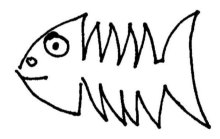

X-ray Fish

X-ray Fish

**Benefits: stretches your neck, opens your chest,
releases tightness from your upper back**

Lie on your back on the ground while looking up at the sky.
Make sure your legs and feet are touching.
Tuck your elbows in by your ribs or the sides of your body.
Roll back on your head, lifting your chest or heart to the sky
while pressing your elbows into the ground.
Gently roll forward with your head to lie back flat on the ground.

Yy

Yak

Yak

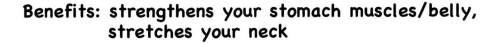

Benefits: strengthens your stomach muscles/belly, stretches your neck

Kneel on the ground with your knees under your hips and your hands under your shoulders like a table.
Keep your back and neck in one straight line, looking at the ground beneath you.
Drop your chin to your chest then look up to the sky.
Repeat again as many times as you like.
Make a Yak sound.

Zz

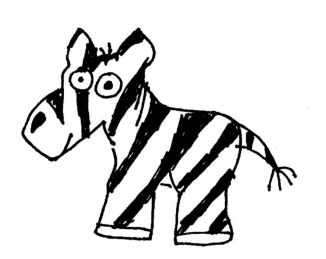
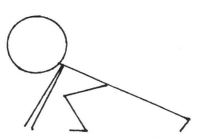

Zebra

Zebra

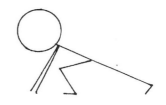

**Benefits: stretches your legs, strengthens your
stomach muscles/belly**

Kneel on the ground with your knees under your hips and your hands
under your shoulders like a table.
Bring your right knee forward to your chest with your knee off the ground.
Repeat bringing you left knee forward to your chest
with your knee off the ground.
Make a zebra sound.
Is a zebra black with white stripes or white with black stripes?

SPECIAL ADDITION

ALTERNATIVE ANIMAL POSES OR POSTURES (ASANAS)

The following are a group of alternative animal poses or postures (asanas) which can be used in place of the ones previously given for a particular letter of the alphabet. For the letter c and cat you can use camel, cow, or crane as illustrated and described as follows or feel free to come up with your own. Be creative!

Bb

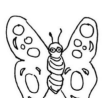

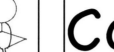

Butterfly

Benefits: stretches lower back,
        opens up the hips and chest

Sit on the ground and bring your feet together
letting your knees drop open to the side.
Clasp your hands around your toes and press your
feet together.
Push your hips forward and lift your chest to the
sky holding onto your toes.
Rock your knees in and out--flapping your wings
to fly.

Cc

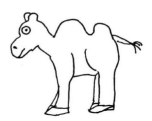

Camel

Benefits: opens up the back, frees your chest, and
        stretches your shoulders.

Begin kneeling on your knees--knees two fists apart.
Push up your hips so you are standing tall on your
knees with arms by your side. Place your hands on
your lower back and lift your chest to the sky. Keep
pushing hips, moving forward as you lift your chest
and draw your shoulders back and down. See if you
can drop your hands and touch your feet while arching your back. Hold for 5-10 deep breaths and
release. Forward with chin to chest to knees and arms
by your side (mouse).

Cc

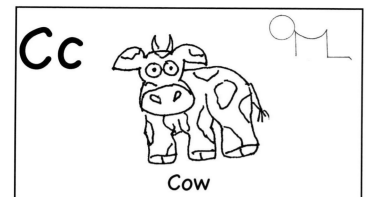

Cow

Benefits: works the spine, reduces tension in the back, increases blood flow.

Kneel on the floor--knees under your hips and hands under your shoulders like a table. With elbows straight, look up and lift your chin away from your chest letting belly button drop toward the floor and inhale. Come back to the table position.

Cc

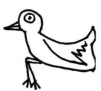

Crane

Benefits: strengthens the arms, upper body and stomach muscles, improves your balance.

Stand tall with feet slightly apart--not touching. Squatting up and down bending your knees to warm them up. Squat down with hands in prayer in front of your heart. Place hands firmly on the ground and spread your fingers. Lean forward into your hands. Lift your heels and rise up on your toes. Keep putting more of your body weight into hands until you can fly your feet off the floor.

Dd

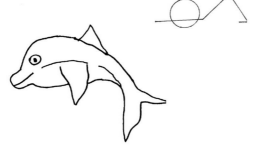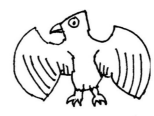

Dolphin

Benefits: strengthens the upper body,
stretches the legs.

Come on to all fours, hands under shoulders/ knees under hips--like a table. Drop your elbows to the floor and clamp your hands together, keeping elbows under your shoulders. Curl your toes under and press your hips up to the sky straightening your legs while resting on your forearms. Lift one leg up behind toward the sky to flap your flipper.

Ee

Eagle

Benefits: strengthens the legs, frees the shoulders, opens up the upper back.

Stand tall, feet together with arms by your side. Take your arms out to your shoulder spreading your wings. Cross your right arm over your left one at your elbows then wrap your right hand around your left arm, bringing your palms together. Shift your weight to your right foot, lift your left foot and try to wrap your left foot behind the back of your right calf, balancing on your right leg only. Look straight ahead and try toe hold for 10 breathes. Repeat on the other side.

Ff

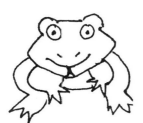

Frog

Benefits: stretches and strengthens ankles, calves, and toes.

Kneel on your floor, knees under hips--two fists width apart. Hands on the floor by your knees. Curl your toes under. Push back with your hands, lifting your bum off the floor. Hop up and down and "Rippet" like a frog.

Gg

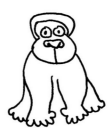

Gorilla

Benefits: frees the upper and middle back, stretches arms/shoulders and legs (hamstring).

Stand tall, feet slightly apart with knees lined up with your feet. Take a breathe and lean forward from hips grab your toes or step on your hands palms up. Press your feet into the ground or hands and pull with your arms.
Make a Gorilla sound.

ANIMAL SALUTATION (Version A)

Move from one animal to the next in this order. Repeat as many times as your like in this mini "Vinyasa" (set sequence or order) flow.

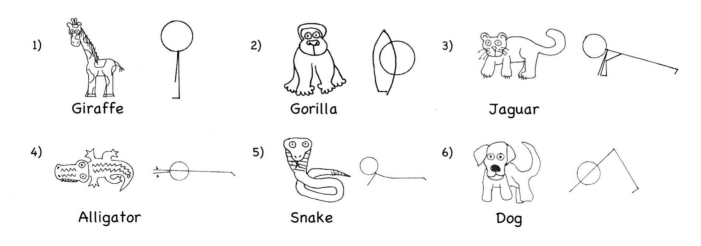

1) Giraffe

2) Gorilla

3) Jaguar

4) Alligator

5) Snake

6) Dog

AUTHOR/ILLUSTRATOR'S BIOGRAPHY
Elizabeth C. Kawecki (known as "Lizzy") M.A., President/Director of Y Yoga Inc.
RYT/IYT/EKYTT (Level 1)/YC/PT/PFI/PRES/CFS

Studied and practiced Kripalu, Ashtanga, Vinyasa, Bikram and Integrative Yoga in Hawaii, California, Brazil and and Florida. Highly athletic individual who discovered yoga after a serious scuba diving accident in 1993 which left her paralyzed on one side of her body, dyslexic, effected her speech and cognitive skills and impaired her balance and coordination. Yoga transformed her life, allowing Lizzy to participate in activities she loved that no one thought she would be able to do again such as: walk without assistance or brace, run, bike, play tennis, golf, surf, hike and kayak. December 2000 completed the Honolulu Marathon. Since then has run several nationally recognized Marathons (LaSalle Chicago, Marine Corp, Honolulu Marathon again 2008) and 1/2 marathons (Disney, Mardi Gras, Outback Classic, AIA, Jacksonville Bank, New Las Vegas, ING Georgia); in addition to several adventure races. In 2006 completed the International Riga 1/2 marathon in Lativa, former Soviet Republic; in addition to teaching "Kids Yoga" at the International School of Latvia (187 students from 25 different nationalities) which sparked the book. As an Integrative Yoga Therapy Teacher, registered with the Yoga Alliance, she offers one-on-one classes and individual therapy sessions. Her classes combine the traditional Hatha Yoga styles for all ages and levels of fitness and practices for: general wellness, rehabilitation, athletic conditioning, weight loss and stress reduction. In addition to being a Certified Pilate Instructor, Personal Trainer, Post Rehabilitation Exercise Specialist, Children Fitness Specialist, Lizzy created and developed specialty classes: Beach Yoga, Aqua Yoga, and Kids Yoga at the Montessori School and McArthur YMCA on Amelia Island in Florida. Very active in a number of charities and non-profit organizations inspiring others to fulfill their highest aspirations.